The Ultimate guide To Starting Your Own Dialysis Unit

BANJI AWOSIKA

PREFACE

My name is Banji Awosika. My father and every one of his siblings had hypertension. At the time I was deciding my career path he had lost a sibling due to complications of hypertension. I had always known I wanted to help people and my dad due to my academic quests, saw the potential for me to become a doctor. After a few years in med school, I left for a year to improve my financial situation. I went to work in London, UK as a cab driver. I actually fell in love with medicine after I left it for a while. I had missed it so much and realized that this what I was actually called to do. Taking care of and servicing the needs of people, as well as educating and showing them how to get healthier, lessening, and eventually eliminating the need for medication. I found that I was very passionate about this, especially the rewarding aspect of hearing from the families of patients that I'm caring for, their wins and testimonies of how they've improved their health by implementing the suggestions that I've made during our time together with their family member, who was actually my patient. This actually blessed the socks off of me. The whole idea is to create ambassadors of this message from the patients to the staff to my colleagues. And in so doing to be able to improve various things.

One of these things that is very important to me is improving the life of my fellow physicians, my colleagues, by illuminating a pathway for them to have a better lifestyle, as I have learned to have. To improve their ability to do things with their loved ones that hitherto they have not been able to do - at least, not in enough quantity as well as quality - because of the lack of adequate passive income. Being able to stop exchanging precious hours for dollars is a quest that I have been put on, and showing people, especially my colleagues, how to do so has become a very strong passion of mine. I aim to impact as many nephrologists, and for that matter other physicians, specialists, and primary care physicians alike, by illuminating a different mindset that can result in a better quality of life. This book is indeed meant for all nephrologists, especially those who already have up to 50 patients receiving dialysis in various dialysis units that want to solve the challenge of not having enough passive income streams and change their consulting every day in the hospital and clinic from a need to a want, and have enough time to do things that they love to do with their loved ones instead. Let's get started.

Banji Awosika 08-Oct-2016

TABLE OF CONTENTS

CHAPTER ONE

Why Become A Nephrologist?

Why become a doctor?

There are various reasons why to become a doctor. Some of my great reasons include, I wanted to help people. Other great reasons include: Wanting to impact my family members who had a tendency towards certain diseases. Another great reason was, I wanted to find answers to all health problems and another noble reason was, I wanted to create a better life for me and my family. Some reasons are suboptimal including "I want to make a lot of money" or "I wanted to be a person with authority". Another suboptimal reason will be, "I wanted to prove myself to my family" or "I wanted to impress my childhood friends". Believe it or not, these are all reasons why some people become doctors. The reason why you become a doctor impacts your overall approach as a doctor, your success as a doctor and the care you provide.

Why go the route of internal medicine?

There are various disciplines in medicine and various tracks. You can go the track of medicine itself, be a clinical practitioner or you can go into clinical research, or actually go the track of being a clinician in the pharmaceutical industry. Now as the physician, you can go down the track of medicine, or obstetrics and gynecology, surgery, pediatrics. If you chose to go down the track of medicine you could go into family practice. You can go into internal medicine. You can go into emergency room medicine. And if you went the route of internal medicine there are various specialties you could now seek to pursue.

The question now becomes what is your motivation? What motivates you to go down the route of internal medicine? For many it may be simply the thrill of diagnosing disease, of discussing with colleagues.

Why specialize?

Various reasons to specialize includes creating a niche for yourself. Creating and impacting the doctors in the community is also very important. Providing a better life for yourself and your family can also be a good reason. Further knowledge acquisition should lead to you becoming more, which leads you doing more and ultimately leads to you having more. The tendency is for you to impact a smaller population of patients much more intensely as a specialist.

Why specialize as a nephrologist?

What was your motivation to be a doctor? Most commonly, it's usually a personal story of things hitting very close to home. That tends to be a very common reason why people tend to specialize in something like nephrology. However, another very common reason is with nephrology you still get to see the whole patient, but on a deeper level or a more focused level. And of course, to create a better life for you and your family, those are very important reasons. And the apparent paucity of nephrologists can also be a motivating factor for people to specialize in nephrology.

Why super specialize in the subspecialty field of nephrology?

There are various ways to super specialize in nephrology. You can go the route of transplant nephrology, or interventional nephrology or Hypertension. One of the reasons why I subspecialized, would be to provide more comprehensive care for my patients. Another reason is, again, to further enhance your knowledge. Because when you acquire more knowledge, you become more, and you're able to do more and have more. I will continue alluding to this fact throughout this book. Adding more value to myself gives me more ability to add to others. Likelihood of success increases when you do massive action. And the likelihood of you doing this increases when you acquire more knowledge.

Paucity of nephrologists

The most common reason for kidney disease is diabetes and this is followed by high blood pressure. The most common reasons for diabetes and high blood pressure is the wrong lifestyle. Burden of disease emanating from chronic diseases is creating demand, a high demand because of the need for many health services. Nephrology services are in very low supply compared to the need for nephrologists, and this paucity is much worse in the third world countries than the first world countries.

Is a nephrologist busier than other doctors?

Your business in any field of medicine is determined, really, by you. In nephrology, there's multitude of potential revenue streams; you can go down each one and be very busy doing them yourself, or the smarter way to do things is to empower other doctors who go down the different, single paths, in which case you'll be less busy. Another approach would be to stay by yourself and go down one or two paths, and also be less busy. Most nephrologists belong to groups, which affords more division of labor - in which case, they'll be less busy. Most of the other doctors in general are in solo or small groups, as opposed to most nephrologists that are in larger groups; so they tend to be busier than most nephrologists are. This is the end of chapter one. For the next chapter, we'll be discussing the academic versus the non-academic setting in nephrology.

CHAPTER TWO

Academic versus Non-Academic Setting

Nephrology fellowship rotations

Nephrology fellowship training can occur in various settings. This may occur in a setting of an academic university owned faculty. Or it may occur in privately owned groups who act as faculty in the hospital, or they may be hybrids of these two models. Depending on the setting, it could be very clinically-based or very researched-based. Another thing that determines the type of nephrology fellowship you undergo would be the ancillary service that are available. Are there vascular surgeons to help with placement of temporary dialysis catheters? Are there interventional radiologists to do the kidney biopsies? Is there a very comprehensive laboratory structure with microscopy to evaluate urine specimens? Are there other allied specialists like endocrinologists, or rheumatologists, or hematologists to brainstorm with the diagnosis of and care of patients? The rotations are a mixture of the consult rotation, transplant nephrology, research rotation and dialysis rotation.

Various tracks as a nephrologist

This is influenced by the type of faculty that trained you. Clinical nephrologist will also be influenced by a clinical nephrologist in an academic vs a non-academic setting. Now you may decide to go down the track of a clinical nephrologist in an academic setting or a non-academic setting. Again, this is influenced by the type of faculty that trained you and what quality of life you want to have. Joining a busy group with 100% nephrology, or less than 100% nephrology also determines how busy you will be and your quality of life. Joining a modern specialty group is also a different track that can be taken. Again, they may have 100% nephrology for you, or less than 100% nephrology where you are doing nephrology along with internal medicine. Another track to take would be the pharmaceutical industry route. Otherwise super specializing such as intervention nephrology, or transplant nephrology may be the track taken. And of course working as an employee of the hospital is another option. All these various option that have been listed determine your quality of life and how busy you'll be, to some extent, determines the potential revenue that can be generated.

What type of city do you want to live in?

This influences your decision as to the track taken. If you're okay with a rural setting, this increases your revenue generating potential. But remember in this setting it is less likely that you have allied specialists, so you end up doing more than what you'll do in the inner city where there are more allied specialists. In the more urban city setting there's obviously less potential for revenue generation. The likelihood is that you join a group of nephrologists, and you are more likely to lose certain skills gained during your training because of allied specialists, such as interventional radiologists and the vascular surgeon.

Mental Masturbation

Mental masturbation. This refers to the dependence on the feel good hormones released when you derive pleasure from things. Discussing with peers and trainees may be more important to you than seeing patients and generating revenue as this leads to the release of this feel good hormone and you thrive on this. Certain individuals will thrive on the significance afforded them in the role of "know-it-all about a particular field." The uncertainty of the real world outside the academic world may be daunting. And some prefer the comfort of the world they have come to know during their nephrology training. The certainty of the academic world may be further affirmed by increased improved quality of life.

Hybrid models

Hybrid models of practice combine the benefits of various models, noted above. Advantages also include reducing the disadvantages of each one by the advantages of the different ones. It tends to attract more doctors which makes them easier to recruit into these settings of the hybrid model.

What motivates you as a nephrologist?

Motivation differs between doctors and is influenced by various things including:

- the type of training setting in terms of faculty, academic versus non-academic setting
- type of place of training
- personal upbringing
- experience of the physician
- Level of self-development.

These are all factors that affect the motivation of a nephrologist or as a doctor for that matter, in general.

Medicine. Art or science or both?

Traditional medicine teaches the science of the practice of medicine. The art of it is not taught, it is actually caught. Today it's more important to develop relationships with your patients than being smart enough to know everything about the disease they have, and treating them based on fantastic knowledge. The art of the practice of medicine results in effective communication and rapport with your patient such that they learn to trust you and trust your opinion. Even if you're not the smartest doctor, having mastered the art of medicine you have a lot of leeway to either enlist the help of other doctors or find out more about the disease and become resourceful in your management of the patient. The best combination is knowing the art and the science of medicine, so developing a good relationship with the patient, in order to communicate effectively with the patient, and being able to manage the patients very well.

This brings us to the end of chapter two. In the next chapter we'll be discussing whether to join a group or not.

CHAPTER THREE

Join A Group or Not

Are you an entrepreneur or a technician?

I read an interesting book called The E-Myth; it delves into this question and it elaborates upon it very eloquently. The myth of the entrepreneur essentially states that, "If I can work as a clinician, as a doctor, or any other service provider or technician, I can provide the services and run the business that provides the service." This will always be a myth, because you can provide the service doesn't mean that you can run the business that provides the service.

You increase your chance of success by self-improvement, learning how to run the business that provides the service. Unfortunately, the training for providing the service does not include the training needed to run the business that provides the service. Persistence is definitely much more important than talent, and with the right mindset – growth mindset, you can learn the business that provides the service.

Do you work well with people?

Team playing is important to achieve success. Learning to work smarter and not harder is also very important for quality of life, and actually achieving success. A part of working smarter is working well within a team. Great book was written by Patrick Lencioni refers to The Five Dysfunctions of a Team and this includes

- Absence of trust,
- Which leads to fear of conflict with artificial harmony.
- This leads to a lack of commitment
- this in turn results in the avoidance of accountability with low standards
- Ultimately results in inattention to results.

Being able to recognize this and develop a game plan to resolve these issues and reverse them leads to much improved success of a team.

5 Dysfunctions of a team

As noted above, the ability to be able to trust your team members and become more vulnerable, and open with your team members leads to an ability to engage in healthy debate without the fear of conflict. Healthy debate without the fear of conflict leads to the ability to commit better. When you enforce clarity and closure as a result of being able to engage in debate and not fear conflict. When you are able to commit to the decision made then you're able to confront difficult issues, and hold each other accountable and raise your standards. And this results in better attention to results and focus on outcomes.

Select your group carefully

Like in marriage the right spouse is very important and you have to look for a group that will complement you, like the right spouse will. Find out what their core values are, what their culture is. Do they align with your core values and the culture you'd want to adopt in your practice? Look at the fruit they have. Have there been court cases? Do they have a good reputation in the community they serve? Have they lots of good will in the community that they serve? Aim to meet the family of the members of the group. You can tell a lot about individuals by the kind of family that they have. Always engage legal counsel to discuss fully the contract you'll be signing with them.

Pros and cons of a solo nephrologist

As the founder of my group, I can tell you firsthand the pros and cons of a solo nephrologist. Some of the pros include:

- No need to be considerate of the thoughts and egos of other doctors.

- The staff learning the ways of only one provider which may theoretically lead to less confusion.

- Smaller and more contained operation.

Some of the cons include:

- Revenue lost during any vacation taken or any coverage by other doctors.

- Nobody to brainstorm with regarding clinical issues.

- Trading dollars for hours.

- Expansion is much slower.

- On-call every night until you have coverage.

- Having to form systems for operation of the clinic.

Pros and cons of starting a group.

Starting a group, there are certain pros and cons. Pros include:

- You get to choose the type of model the group will follow.

- As founder you get to set the culture.

- As founder, you get to set the pace.

- You also leverage the goodwill you have accumulated.

Some cons include;

- You work hard to expand by providing service to more people to accommodate added doctors such that you have enough business to keep them busy.

- You have expenses added to the bottom line as they join, sometimes going without a salary in order for the doctors to be paid.

- When wrong doctors are invited to join and isn't a good fit, you get the blame for this disruption by your colleagues and other partners.

Pros and cons of being in group.

The pros of being in a group include

- Shared calls.

- Join already formed systems that work.

- Clinical focus with no need to be mixed with administration.

- Discussion about cases are encouraged.

- You ride the tail of the goodwill of the group.

- You enjoy the strengths of your various partners.

Cons include;

- Having to conform to ways of a new group.

- Effecting change is more difficult because the group has to be sold on the idea.

- Working with staff trained a certain way and having to re-train them to do things your way as well.

This brings us to the end of chapter three. The next chapter we'll be delving into the revenue streams of the nephrologist.

CHAPTER FOUR

Revenue Streams as a Nephrologist

Earning capacity of specialists versus primary care physician

Earning capacity of doctors depend on the doctor and to a less extent on whether or not he's a specialist or a primary care physician. Having said that, to some extent, the capacity to earn is influenced by the structure of your practice. So certain factors become important including:

- Is the practice procedure-based, in which case the doctors have a higher earning capacity.
- Doctors whose procedures don't require hospitalization have a higher earning capacity.
- Doctors whose procedures require hospitalization get paid very well by the hospital.

Primary care physicians are not dependent on the specialists for a referral, as opposed to the specialist who is dependent upon the primary care physician for a referral.

So, in this situation, the primary care physician has more leeway with the procedures and a lack of accountability, as opposed to the specialist who does remain accountable to the primary care physician. This may be a good thing or a bad thing. We all need some accountability but we don't need to be micromanaged.

The average nephrologist

The average nephrologist earns their revenue by typical evaluation and management by patients seen in the clinic, as well as in the hospital, as well as in the dialysis clinic. Occasionally they also have the revenue stream of the medical directorship of dialysis units. These average nephrologists tend to outsource all other services. They tend to attend conferences that are focused on nephrology probably every two to five years. On average they have three to four members of staff in the office and when in a group, typically have three staff members per nephrologist.

Revenue streams of the nephrologists in academic settings

In academic settings, the nephrologists have the same revenue stream as the average nephrologist but, in addition, they also have the revenue streams that result from:

- Research grants

- Education stipends

- Pharmaceutical Talks

- Speaking engagements

Revenue streams of nephrologists in a non-academic setting

In a non-academic setting, revenue streams may also include the same things as noted above in the average nephrologist and the nephrologist in their clinic setting. But in addition, they tend to outsource the services a little less hence there may be an in-house laboratory, - in-house ultrasound services. Medication administration such as intravenous iron erythropoietin simulating agents. The less commonly employed revenue streams in non-academic settings include.

Less commonly employed revenue streams in non-academic settings

In addition to the services provided by nephrologists in a non-academic setting, a few less commonly employed revenue streams will include:

- Providing dialysis services

- Vascular access centers.

- Phase one and phase two clinical trials/research centers.

Medical directorship

As a nephrologist, the medical director usually operates in the setting of a dialysis unit. It usuall involves things that as a nephrologist you typically would do in the dialysis unit, but a few othe things are done as well.

The medical director tends to supply the unit with patients as well, although this is not part of th job description of the medical director There will be patients referred from practicing nephrologis in the community. Unfortunately, these dialysis directorships come with very restrictiv covenants. Medical directorship is akin to leasing a nice house or nice car as this shifts one's focu away from the need for ownership. There is a complex formula used to derive the medical directc fees.

The right mindset

Mindset acts like a gate to opportunities

Mindset refers to the preferred mindset, which is a growth mindset versus the less preferre mindset which is the fixed mindset. But the growth mindset essentially allows you to approac things without the negativity of limiting thoughts or a fragile sense of belonging or letting peopl define you. Here you are able to extract the pearls from the chaff and you avoid the possibility c group think since the brilliance of the individual who's reverred and talented and whom unlimite faith has been placed is not in play. People with a growth mindset want to open discussic depending on collective thoughts and they welcome critics from the team.

So, a fixed mindset denotes a mindset where one requires success without effort, typically findin failure absolutely unbearable, instead always looking for someone else to blame. This is differe from the growth mindset which refers to the ability to, not only learn appropriately, but also seek to enjoy, and get the most out of the learning process, as opposed to basking only in attainment c a title, and its attendant stigma. You're more likely to have your mind thrive by having a growth mindset.

The tendency is with the right growth mindset, it gets wide open, encouraging and attracting lots of opportunities. With the wrong mindset, the gate is closed, and opportunities are repelled, and opportunities pass you by.

This brings us to the end of chapter four. Next chapter will be delving into the dialysis unit.

CHAPTER FIVE

The Dialysis Unit

Types of dialysis units by modality

Dialysis involves the clearance of blood of waste products, usually cleared by the kidneys, especially urea, potassium, phosphorus, sodium, and chloride. This can be done by passing blood through the dialyzer, in which case it's referred as hemodialysis, or using peritoneal lining as well as capillary walls of vessels in the peritoneum, and the filter aligned for transfer of waste from blood to fluid in the cavity, which is then referred as peritoneal dialysis. Hemodialysis can be in center or part of a home therapy, which clears to be home hemodialysis on off-channel in center. PD can be automated using a cycler - CCPD - or ambulatory and manually - CAPD.

Types of dialysis in its groups

Dialysis unit groups are usually based on number of units in the chain of dialysis units. Largest unit groups refer to as the LDU include groups like fresenius and davita and certain other groups, medium-sized groups and small-sized groups depending on the number of dialyses in the chain

Capital outlay of the multimodality dialysis unit

Capital needed for putting together dialysis unit is very variable, depending on various factors. There could be dialysis unit which is single-modality, or just pure PD, or just purely in-center hemodialysis, or just purely home hemodialysis, or just purely nocturnal in-center. - It could be a multimodality which would be a combination of the above mentioned signal modalities. Other factors that would affect the capital outlay would include leasing versus buying of machines, leasing versus owning the building, staff structure, water system, the number of in-center stations, the number of in-center shifts. These all affect the capital outlay.

The corporate world of dialysis

This is a very complex world where though the nephrologists are the lifeline of the dialysis unit, they do not make the important decisions in the dialysis unit. It's usually headed by a non-nephrologist, very savvy businessmen who successfully manage the nephrologists and their dialysis patients. and usually runs the dialysis unit. Typically, joint ventures are done with nephrologists with the result of sharing relatively small profit margins because of the operations and administration model

Revenue streams from providing dialysis services and dialysis equipments and also now acquiring nephrology practices, and more recently MSOs with primary care practices, make up some of the revenue streams of the corporate dialysis centers.

What do the dialysis patient complain about?

The dialysis patients complaints depend on various factors. Education pre-dialysis is a very important factor.

Type of access, stuff to do with is also a very important factor. The length of time of nephrology care before dialysis also affects the complaints of the patients. The type of dialysis, and the social support structure the dialysis patient has, as well as their comorbidities also affects their complaints. Complaints include, but not limited to:

1. non-communication from care providers in center.

2. not seeing a nephrologist frequently.

3. pain at the access site.

4. length of time on dialysis.

5. number of days per week of dialysis.

6. temperature in the unit.

7. waiting to get on the machine.

8. any change in technicians or RNs, caring for them.

9. cramping.

10. fullness of belly before the belly is drained.

11. constipation.

12. abdominal pain on draining.

13. abdominal pain on filling.

Policy And Procedures

Policy and procedure is for human dialysis units proprietary documents. They're actually quite standard for multimodality centers, and essentially contain every aspect of the operations of a multimodality dialysis center. This is in place so that the employees understand their role, and how they function as a team. QAPI is the cumulative effect of policy and procedures, and the whole operation is essentially reviewed monthly, covering all aspects and all roles in the dialysis unit.

Joint Ventures

Joint ventures are becoming more common between the dialysis chains and the local nephrologists. They can also be agreements between the hemodialysis chains and hospitals. Joint ventures are typically the way the nephrologists acquire equity ownership in dialysis units. Equity ownership currently range from 20% to 49%. Joint ventures with large dialysis organization has multiple advantages and lots of disadvantages. Certain advantages include management which is essentially a system that's been put in place in various other dialysis units by the large dialysis organization. And the nephrologist actually just provides the patients and acts as medical director. However, one major disadvantage of this is essentially the fact that there is less chance of an exit strategy with the sale of the unit if the joint venture occurs with the large dialysis organization, as there's no one else to sell it to. Another issue is the EBITDA of the joint venture in question. Upon a sale, it essentially does not allow for the goodwill that has been accumulated in the fair market value during the potential sale. Essentially, the joint ventures have occurred most beneficially with the medium-size and small-size dialysis organizations because this can now be sold to the next tier, in which case, a lot of your capital outlay is recovered in multiples.

This brings us to the end of chapter five. In the next chapter we'll be delving into the lifestyle as a nephrologist.

CHAPTER SIX

Lifestyle as a Nephrologist

Lifestyle as a Physician

As a physician, lifestyle is dictated by various factors such as:

- One's priorities in terms of family, motivation, community.

- The specialists versus primary, and this definitely affects both tracks in various ways as has already been elucidated.

- A solo practitioner verses a group, a vision that belongs to a group. Again, this has already been discussed.

- Rural setting versus city.

- Academic versus non-academic.

- Clinic-based nephrologists versus a hospital predominant nephrologists versus both.

All these factors definitely affects one's lifestyle as a physician. But no matter what category you fit into, your lifestyle is ultimately dictated by you and what your priorities are, what you motivation is. As a rule, aim to work smarter, not necessarily harder.

Lifestyle as a Specialist.

A specialist's lifestyle is influenced by similar factors to the physician including one's priorities motivation.

- Academic versus nonacademic.

- Rural versus city.

- Group versus solo.

As was mentioned for a physician as a specialist, your priorities really influence your lifestyle. And there are various ways and collaborations that can be struck to improve one's lifestyle as a specialist. However, this definitely comes, sometimes at a price, such as a price in terms of a cut in salary or a cut in revenue, or a cut in time in order to boost revenue, with more time being diverted to generating revenue. It's actually trading hours for dollars.

As a nephrologist, different paces can be taken.

As a nephrologist, you may choose to be fast-paced, by doing things such as:

- Multiple hospitals being consulted in with an increase in inpatient care, especially in the intensive care unit.

- Multiple clinics, where patients are seen in the outpatient setting at multiple locations.

- Multiple dialysis patients in multiple dialysis units. So as a nephrologist, I was going to 25 different dialysis units and seeing patients once a week on my own prior to having my current partners join me and nurse practitioner.

- Hybrid. Various hybrid model of the above mentioned situations.

Slow-paced nephrologist usually occurs in the setting of the group practice where time can be better planned. In this situation there are:

- Less patients to be seen per doc than in the solo practice.

- Less tendency to be in various places on a daily basis.

Certain hybrids model exists where the certain period of the month are fast-paced and other period of the month are less fast-paced.

Lifestyle Dependent on Path Taken

Various paths can be taken as a nephrologist, and this is strong determinant of the lifestyle that would be the case. Easiest path is that where the nephrologist works in pharmaceutical companies. He has a much better quality of life. It's actually pretty decent revenue, paid very well by the pharmaceutical companies, and there's less clinical work. Depending on the individual, this can be a good thing or a bad thing. In the case of the academic pathway, the nephrologist act as a supervisor supervising work done by the trainees. That is nephrology fellows. Out patient clinic is usually quite light because of the needs as a supervisor work done by the fellows. Call schedule tends to be much lighter because the calls actually being handled by the fellows with the attending nephrologist being on the call for major issues that the fellows don't feel comfortable handling, which with some of us was almost never.

Non-academic group practice would be next in line in terms of time commitment and quality of life. In this situation, they do see more patients than would be seen by an academic nephrologist. But definitely not as much as would be seen by a non-academic, solo-practice nephrologist.

Inpatient versus Outpatient

Inpatient care is often a busier night on-call but sometimes can be more profitable with less expenses. It's actually function as pure profit. The outpatient care definitely results in much less calls per night when one is on call because generally patients are much more stable in the outpatient setting. More expenses are generated by the clinical staff in order to provide the service in the outpatient setting, which include the back MAs, and the front desk and administration. Lifestyle taking care of more acute inpatients may generally be busier than the more stable outpatient especially since clinical appointment times can be planned to suit one's schedule. Outpatient care can also result in more passive income streams, in which case, you're working smarter and not harder. Most services that are required as part of the management of the patient in the hospital are automatically outsourced to the hospital. However, in the clinic, these outsourcing can be kept to a bare minimum with everything being done in house.

Inpatient heavy in one hospital or light to medium in multiple hospitals.

Lifestyle also dictated by the inpatient distribution. If the nephrologist has high patient census in one hospital, there's less drive time, less walking to the hospital from the car, less walking from the hospital back to the car, and less socializing time. At first looking at this, this may sound like quite trivial issues, however, when you're going to four or five hospitals, these minutes add up to substantial amounts of time and makes the difference between having a busy lifestyle and a not so busy lifestyle. If one is light to medium in multiple hospitals, then again, these factors make a huge difference with more drive time. There's more risk of other slow down issues such as traffic, weather and there's also the need to socialize. There is more time to socialize which is a very necessary part of business, essentially marketing yourself.

The type of hospital is also important because the typical closed intensive care unit results in issues being handled by the intensivist, and this results in less night calls and less need to actually see patients acutely in the hospital at night. Also, of course, patients still occasionally need to be seen by nephrologists at night to initiate dialysis if need be. Small hospitals where the intensive care unit is not closed, and they have less allied specialists. There may be more calls, more need to go to the hospital. Interestingly, at small hospitals, nurses are many times actually more independent than in larger hospitals, which sometimes leads to a better lifestyle for the nephrologist in the small hospital.

Dialysis patients in how many different dialysis units

As a nephrologist, you are affected by various things as noted above. Specifically, number of dialysis units that house your patients is a very strong determining factor because as I noted earlier, at one stage I had my patients were in 25 different dialysis units. This significantly affects your

24

lifestyle. Another factor, refers to the number of visits needed per month. Are you utilizing th service of a nurse practitioner? Do you have partners? These questions are key questions to b answered in order to predict one's lifestyle. Do you have your own dialysis unit that houses mos of your patients? This is a very important question as this significantly affects your lifestyle especially if you're able to position your dialysis unit next to your clinic. Do you have to succuml to a culture of the dialysis unit, which influences the care of your patients, positively o negatively? And another important question that affects one's lifestyle, and affects the care tha you're able to provide as a nephrologist to your patients on dialysis. Does any dialysis staff knov your overall care plan, resulting in less calls, despite communication?

In this case, being in sync with the dialysis team is very important. And this results in better car being given to your patients during dialysis with less calls being made to you after you've left th dialysis unit. If everybody's on the same page and a care plan is in place for the patient, wher everyone is engaged and involved, this leads to much better care, and ultimately, the possibility o making impact on the current mortality rate becomes much more attainable.

This brings us to the end of chapter six. Next chapter we'll be delving into stepping outside the bo: and giving back.

CHAPTER SEVEN

Stepping Outside the Box and Giving Back

Uncommon Revenue Streams

Less common revenue streams includes research. In this case, this can be done in conjunction with a partner who's already a clinical researcher, or research centers conducting research with you. And there are different routes for a nephrologists to employ a researcher in your center to conduct research on your unique population of patients. Either way, having a partnership, or equity ownership, in a research center is definitely a much less common revenue stream for the nephrologist. This should, however, be more common as we have a unique set of patients who can be the subjects in several groundbreaking clinical trials that can result in the improvement of their quality of life, and ultimately, mortality.

In-house pharmacy is also another revenue stream that is not very commonly tapped into, but does definitely create another revenue stream.

Providing nephrology services and dialysis services to nursing home facilities is also an area where most nephrologists don't venture into, but definitely fits under the umbrella of uncommon revenue streams.

Be motivated by providing excellent care, not money

Aim to add value to your patients while caring for them. Tend to over promise, commit, and then over deliver. Another awesome approach to care is exchange in abundance. Exchange in abundance actually provides services that by far outweigh the revenue generated from the service. Be motivated by a cause, a cause higher than money. This is very important because money is actually a very low motivator. When you find the strong enough WHY and you're able to identify with a cause beyond actual money, the tendency to stay aligned with this cause and motivated is very high. This is especially the case if it's done as a group where everyone is in alignment and ar motivated by the same higher cause. Aim to add more value to yourself by reading in and aroun your field and engage in self development courses or seminars. Become more this month than yo were last month, or this year than you were last year, because once you become more as a resul of knowing more, you tend to do more. Once you do more, as a result of becoming more, you ten to have more, so be, do, have.

Pass on your Knowledge to the Next Generation of Doctors

Learn more with the intent to teach more. Once you are able to do this, you essentially becom more and the tendency is that you'll do more as noted above. In this case, teach everyone wh comes into your sphere. A nephrologist should aim to impact everyone. Let them always leave yo more knowledgeable than they were before they met you. Write down your experiences, you opinions, your moments of revelation, your reflections, and let people learn from your mistake and successes. It's amazing how much priceless information lies in graveyards today because ver few people took time to document their experiences in life that form treasure boxes, and whe given to the right person or planted in the right mind results in amazing creativity, amazin innovation, amazing breakthroughs. Be encouraged to pass on your information to the nex generation of physicians, to the next generation of nurses, to the next generation of healthcar providers, so that as a whole, people can benefit from you - both the providers and the recipients Helping doctors avoid the pitfalls you fell into, or people you know fell into is priceless. If yo had an opportunity to get to take a shortcut to where you are now, wouldn't you be forever full o gratitude to the person who provided the short cut for you - that's what mentorship is about. So b a mentor.

Provide Comprehensive Care

Look for ways to exchange in abundance as noted above, and provide care to the patients' benefit and convenience, essentially, cater to the patient. Take responsibility for the patient getting needed tests, needed procedures, done in such a way that it's convenient for him. Most convenient ways to have all the services that you would typically outsource, all under your roof. You should have patients able to come in and go through a one-stop shop. Trust me, they appreciate this. This is especially the case when they're receiving dialysis either at home or in-center where their dialysis takes up many hours of their week. They're able to cut down drive time and planning time and all of the logistics that are involved with having to see their doctor at a different clinic site, go to the access center at a different clinic site, do an ultrasound, do lab-work - they will do all this under one roof and avoid being hospitalized. This is indeed comprehensive care.

Anything Referred Can Be Done In-House

Outsourcing sometimes saves companies money. There's no doubt about this. It all depends on the volume of units to be outsourced. If the volumes of units to be outsourced are significant enough, keeping them in-house may generate substantial passive income for the nephrologist. Many services exist such as:

- Lab tests.

- Ultrasound services.

- Intravenous iron administration

- Subcutaneous erythropoietin stimulating agents.

- Sleep studies

- Dialysis provision.

- Vascular Access Care.

- In-house pharmacy.

These are some of the services that are typically outsourced. There are others that have not been elucidated, but this is a pretty comprehensive list.

Aim to Keep Patients Out of the Hospital

Most common reasons why dialysis patients are admitted to the hospital has already been discussed earlier. Some of the reasons include volume overload with congestive heart failure access dysfunction, and other reasons that are unrelated to hemodialysis such as chest pain or back pain. Having access to a dialysis unit where you are able to be dialyzed at a moment's notice, i very important for the dialysis patient. So as a nephrologist, having access to this type of dialysi unit will help you keep your patient's out of the hospital, as patients don't need to be admitted - a they currently are being admitted through the emergency room. This is because patient need dialysis today even though patient is presenting to the emergency room with problems that don' require admission. Also, having access to a Vascular Access Center, where they are able to take care of emergent procedures such as dysfunctional catheters and dysfunctional dialysis accesse that need to be declotted, or peritoneal catheters that need to be changed also results in th avoidance of an unnecessary hospital stay. This is beneficial both in terms of cost to the variou insurance companies, or more important in terms of quality of life of the patient. It is a fact that b being admitted to the hospital, patient is at risk for iatrogenic causes of increased morbidity, a well as mortality. They are also at risk for going through the unnecessary trauma of the whol experience of being hospitalized. The waiting in the emergency room, the waiting to get a bed in the inpatient setting, the waiting to be taken care of while an inpatient, the waiting to being teste and diagnosed and seeing the doctor, the waiting to be dialyzed, and ultimately, the waiting to b discharged. If you are able to provide your patients access to these facilities, you should make th emergency room aware of this, thus preventing the need for hospitalizations. The emergency room physician actually appreciates this very much, because they know as well that admitting the patients just to be dialyzed, or to do things that could be better done outpatient, is a very painful decision for them to make as well.

Give Back to the Community

Provide education as a nephrologist, for your community, especially the at-risk population. At-risk education programs can be put together to this effect. And this way, you're giving back in terms of time, talent and treasure. When giving back, aim to remain compliant with the regulations of healthcare, in our case the CMS, and the restrictions imposed on what we can and cannot do without being paralyzed by them. Remember, ultimately, what comes from the heart gets to the heart and if your heart is to help people, they will be helped, without you necessarily getting in trouble for helping.

END CHAPTER

We've been able to go through some very pertinent points, starting with discussing why one should become a nephrologist, and then delving into the differences between the academic and the non-academic setting. This, in turn, led to us discussing whether or not you should join a group, and then exploring the potential revenue streams as a nephrologist. We then delved into the dialysis unit, discussing that in a more in-depth way, and then we visited the lifestyle as a nephrologist, and finally explored the amazing benefits of stepping outside the box and actually giving back.

Please take action to finally have a three-day work week, or a two-day work week, or even a seven-day work week, but a work week that you have because it's what you want and not necessarily what you need. You would be able to do this now because you now have great passive income streams, and you're finally able to stop having to consult every day in the hospital and clinic, but instead be able to do things you love to do with your loved ones. The first step is to call my office at 407-988-1065 and ask for Ynolandy, and tell her I want to take advantage of Dr. Awosika's "equity ownership in dialysis units," and she will get you all set up.